Strategic Victory Manual for Veterans and their Families

Recover From and Overcome PTSD By Applying These15 Successful Principles Together!

Every day, twenty-two veterans commit suicide. Nine percent of all inmates have served on active duty. Over eight percent of the homeless are veterans. PTSD and other mental illnesses affect families and friends as well.

In this revolutionary Itty Bitty Book, Earl J. Katigbak shows you how to cope with issues veterans face as a family and community.

Apply these simple and effective 15 principles with your veteran and family in order to recover from and claim victory over PTSD.

In this book, you will discover:

- What to do if your veteran becomes suicidal.

- How veterans can re-assimilate into the lives of their children.

- How to find the right therapist.

Pick up a copy of this powerful book today and discover how to heal from PTSD and other issues you and your family may be facing with your veteran.

Your Amazing Itty Bitty®

Veterans Survival Book

15 Keys to Help You & Your Family Deal with PTSD

Earl J. Katigbak

Published by Itty Bitty® Publishing
A subsidiary of S & P Productions, Inc.

Printed in the United States of America

Itty Bitty® Publishing
311 Main Street, Suite D
El Segundo, CA 90245
(310) 640-8885

ISBN: 978-1-931191-07-4

First and foremost, this book is dedicated to the United States of America. My home, the land of my birth, and ultimately, the place of my deepest healing.

This guidebook was intended for families of veterans and for all Americans. Despite our individual political beliefs, it is our responsibility to care for those who sacrifice their lives in defense of this country.

A Word on "Did You Kill Anyone?"

- "Did you kill anyone?"
- "Did any of your buddies die?"
- "Do You Have PTSD?"
- "Do you regret going there?"

Author Alex Horton, from his blog, "The Civilian-Veteran Survival Field Manual," said it best:

> "The questions above make any Veteran cringe, and I've gotten them many times in the past from well-meaning, but tragically unaware people. They are the primary reason I keep my service with some people a secret. It should be common sense to stay away from such flippant, offensive questioning, but our blood-soaked culture doesn't always allow for discreet and respectful questions distanced from the gore of

combat. Yes, those things are true of some people who leave the service. No, it is not any of your business. If we want to talk about those things, we'll bring it up. Until then, loud parties, bars and the break room are hardly appropriate venues to discuss violent death and the philosophy of war."

(Horton, 2011)

Table of Contents

Introduction

Please visit our Itty Bitty Website and learn more about Veteran issues and PTSD.

http://www.ittybittypublishing.com

You can contact Earl by going to:
https://goo.gl/y8m6KZ

Introduction

In this Itty Bitty® Book, you will find 15 simple things you can do help veterans overcome the symptoms of post-traumatic stress. Whether you're family, a friend, co-worker, colleague or church member, knowing how to approach the issues we veterans face can make the difference.

If the veteran in your life is in need of help, get help immediately! Call the Veterans Crisis Line at 1-800-273-8255 and Press 1, or send a text message to 838255 explaining that this veteran you love needs help.

In this book you will learn to identify PTSD and depression, and you will learn how to respond in a swift, yet gentle manner.

Key 1
Gather Information

For the family and friends of veterans, the first
step in helping is to gather information. By
understanding the symptoms of PTSD better, you
can understand the impact that it has on you.
Begin with the four items below to get you
started.

1. Get informed. Education for the whole
   family is vital for your veteran and
   everyone around them.
2. Join a support group or support
   community.
3. Approach your friend or family member
   about individual therapy.
4. Get into couples counseling (for partners
   or spouses) or family counseling.

PTSD affects you, as well as your veteran.
Contact your local Vet Center for help. Vet
Centers are community-based resources that are
there to help. Each center has group, couples and
individual counseling available. Go to
http://www.vetcenter.va.gov/

Effects Of PTSD On Spousal, Romantic And Interpersonal Relationships

- Problems within a marriage or romantic partnership.
- Problems relating to friends and other family members.
- Parenting problems or difficulty getting along with the children.
- Breakdown in functioning within the family.
- Aggression and irrational outbursts of anger toward others.
- Domestic violence or violence toward others.
- Symptoms of depression.
- General feelings of the onset of a nervous breakdown.

Key 2
What To Do If Your Veteran Is Suicidal Or Having An Episode

Every day, twenty-two veterans commit suicide – veterans combined from the wars of Vietnam to the recent wars in Iraq and Afghanistan. Whether or not you know for sure, take every comment about suicide seriously. **Call 9-1-1 if your veteran needs immediate help!**

The following can guide you in helping your veteran who may be contemplating suicide.

1. Take every comment about suicide seriously.
2. Remember: Suicidal behavior is a cry for help
3. Listen without interruption and judgment.
4. Ask: Are you having thoughts of suicide?
5. If the person is suicidal, you cannot leave them alone!
6. Don't keep your warrior's suicidal behavior a secret. Tell someone who may be able to help.
7. **CALL 911** or the Veteran's Crisis Line at **800-273-8255** and **press 1** to speak with a trained professional right away.

Veteran Suicide Warning Signs

You can help a veteran and save his or her life.
Some signs that your veteran may be
contemplating suicide are:

- Feelings of being a burden or that they
  don't belong.
- Significant relationship, financial,
  medical or work-related problems.
- Current or pending disciplinary or legal
  action.
- Alcohol or drug abuse (to include
  prescribed medications).
- Problems with a major life transition
  (e.g., retirement, discharge, divorce, etc.).
- Loss of a unit member or veteran friend.
- Isolation from friends and family.

Key 3
Tips For Avoiding Painful Issues With Your Veteran

In addition to recovering from PTSD, we get requests from many people to talk about it. You may be the 36th person to ask us to talk about our experiences. Resistance or trepidation to speak with you may also come out of the fear that you may project your own feelings and attitudes about what we went through, making about you instead. The following tips should guide you to having positive results when speaking to us.

1. Don't talk to us about politics.
2. Don't be casual with your questions.
3. Don't assume every veteran has PTSD.
4. Don't pretend to understand, or attempt to relate.
5. Don't push us to go to therapy.
6. Don't expect us to talk about it [PTSD] with you.
7. Don't be offended if we don't talk to you about it.
8. Don't give ultimatums.
9. Don't ask about our experiences in a combat zone.

Things To Consider

Post-traumatic stress is complex and very layered. Although you don't have to walk on eggshells, it's important to allow your war fighter space and time to open up.

- Veterans are not spokespeople for your or opposing political beliefs or agendas.
- Tough Love is not recommended as it more than likely will be responded to with aggression or violence.
- Listen without interruption and get rid of interjecting with "but..."

Key 4
Tips For Gently Opening Up Conversation With Your Veteran

Veterans are not asking you to tread lightly. Instead, veterans are asking for space and invitations. Do the following to facilitate and improve communication.

1. Do: Ask your veteran about their buddies.
   a. What were they like?
   b. What funny stories would you like to share?
2. Do: Listen.
   a. Without interruption.
   b. Without judgment or shoulds.
3. Do: Your homework.
   a. Learn more about military culture.
   b. Learn the language.
4. DO: Have an open mind.
   a. Veterans are not brainwashed machines.
   b. Not all veterans are alcoholics.
   c. Veterans look like everyone else.
   d. There aren't millions of homeless veterans.
   e. Veterans are as young as 22 years old.

Sometimes, all your veteran can muster is "I love you."

If you're in a relationship with a veteran with PTSD or traumatic brain injury (TBI), these simple principles will help you in your communication.

- Short & Clear: Have your messages be clear and concise. Too many details can be stressful.
- Give lots of space and time to answer.
- Be okay with silence.

Key 5
Identify Your Personal Feelings and Triggers

When a Soldier, Sailor, Airman, or Marine experiences post-traumatic stress, family and friends are affected as well. The following principles will give you – the family and friends of veterans – a formula to keep your own state of mental balance.

1. Grieve: Give yourself permission to grieve. Your veteran is forever changed just by being in the military. Give yourself a safe space to express the heavy emotions you're facing.
2. Self-Care: Schedule a massage. Pick up a hobby, or take a class.
3. Get back into a routine: Creating schedules and To-Do Lists will create a sense of normalcy and stability.
4. Create a support system. Enlist the help of other family and friends.
5. See a therapist just for you.

Common Reactions to family members with PTSD

Because your loved one may not have overcome the effects of PTSD, you may be indirectly affected in certain ways. Sometimes simple awareness of your own behavior can help you to cope while caring for your warrior. Seek assistance if you experience the following:

- Feel discouraged, alienated, even hurt.
- Neglect your own needs by focusing on caring for your loved one.
- Foregoing activities you once enjoyed because you want to be there for your veteran.
- Feeling angry because PTSD doesn't let your veteran keep a job or because your veteran drinks too much.
- Feelings of loss or depression because your loved one is no longer the same person.

Key 6
Implement Self-Care

Congratulations! You have chosen the mission of
care-giving for your loved one. In order for
you—friends and family— to fully support your
veterans, implementing self-care will allow you
to re-charge and make life easier.

It's time for you to actually do it!

Take care of yourself by:

1. Eating well.
2. Being physically active.
3. Preventing back injury.
4. Getting enough sleep.
5. Preventive health care.
6. Pampering yourself at least twice a
   month.

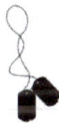

Some Symptoms Of Caregiver Burnout

Be advised: When caregiving for your loved one, your own emotional, physical, and spiritual health will be challenged. The rigors of this mission can lead to fatigue and even burnout. Recognize the symptoms, then apply appropriate self-care counter-measures.

- Emotional and physical exhaustion.
- Excessive use of alcohol and/or sleep medications.
- Irritability.
- Changes in sleep patterns.
- Getting sick more often.

Seek advice and mentoring from your local VA Hospital or Veterans Center to ensure success in your mission as caregiver.

Key 7
How To Re-assimilate Your Veteran Into The Lives Of The Children

Children will react differently to those recently returning home from the warfront, especially depending on their age. Smaller children may cling to the parent who did not deploy. To help during this time, spouses and family can:

1. Gently remind children that, as much as their veteran has changed, so have they.
2. They've had to learn to live without the deployed parent, so they'll need time to get used to him or her again.
3. Let the kids get used to your returning veteran again and let them make the invitation to play.
4. Let the kids know that it's ok for them to share their feelings. Remember that their feelings have nothing to do with mom or dad and vice-versa.
5. Maintain plans and routines.
6. Educate the kids about what PTSD is and that they don't need to fear. Remind them repeatedly that they're ok and that the returning parent will also need their help.

How To Regain Wholeness As A family

You can help your children by explaining how PTSD can affect a family.

- Without going into graphic details, explain why mom or dad behaves that way.
- Remind them that this has nothing to do with them. Let them know that they're not to blame.
- Repeat until they understand.

In addition to what we've just discussed, consider these as well:

- Individual treatment for the children.
- Family therapy.

Key 8
Recruit Help from Other
Family Members

If you are a parent of someone on active duty, reserve components, or a recently discharged veteran, the following should help you have some well-received family time.

1. Give your son or daughter space and allow them to decompress. A quick hello, or a welcome home note will do.
2. Don't ask questions about the war or the military. Often, they just want to come home to my mom and dad and not have to talk about anything.
3. Mom's home cooking.

Tips For Friends & Extended Family

I was happy to see my friends, but even they couldn't understand. Here are a few tips that should help you and your veteran friends.

- Don't ask them about the war, where they were and what happened. Have fun and joke around… a lot!
- Keep offering to take your veteran friend out. Be ok with ninety-nine "No" responses. Eventually there will be a "Yes."
- Bribe them with food. Buffalo wings at Hooters is preferred.
- If your friend has an episode (e.g. gets into a fight, gets irrationally angry), stay calm – and in a peaceful, yet assertive manner, calm them down.
- Treat your friend like a normal human being.

Key 9
Overcome Reasons For Not Getting Help

Obstacles and oppositional feelings may arise
when attempting to get your veteran help. The
following information will help in these
instances:

1. Identify the obstacle and reframe.
   a. What's the excuse?
   b. What positive solutions can I
      offer?
2. Change the environment to dissolve
   defensiveness.
   a. Offer to meet for coffee, or
      barbecue, then ask your veteran
      to make an appointment
   b. Offer a reward, such as the
      movies, after the appointment.
3. Offer a ride to the appointment, or help
   discuss other options.
4. Compare the experience to professional
   sports. Offer examples of athletes getting
   their mental game in order.

Reframe reasons in a calm and gentle way and
your veteran will be more open to going. Stay
calm and persistent. Eventually, your loved one
will seek treatment.

Reasons Veterans May Not Seek Help

- The belief that they can get better on their own.
- Access or obstacles to getting appropriate help.
- Mistrust of therapists or psychiatrists.
- Fear of being seen as weak.
- Fear that PTSD treatments might not work.
- Fear of getting in trouble at work.
- Fear of being labeled or judged.
- Fear that benefits will be affected or they will no longer qualify.

Key 10
Finding The Right Therapist

It's perfectly ok to change therapists if need be. Help your veteran find the right one for them.

1. They're not all doctors, so find one that has experience treating people who've experienced trauma.
2. Try to find one that specializes in effective evidenced-based treatment.
3. If your loved one has insurance outside the VA, call to find out what mental health providers they will pay for. Many of them have lists of providers that they will cover.
4. Ask your veteran's regular doctor for a recommendation.
5. Ask family and friends who they would recommend as well.
6. If your veteran is currently working with someone that doesn't feel like a good fit, ask for someone else. The VA works for you, not the other way around!

Some Signs Of A Good Therapist

A good therapist is one you feel supported by and valued when they listen to you. A good trauma therapist will help your veteran feel empowered and give them the tools to move forward in life. Remember… it's ok to fire your therapist and seek a new one! They are not all the same.

Some Signs of a Good Therapist include:

- Mutual respect.
- Unconditional positive regard.
- Genuine.
- Have firm boundaries, but are not bossy.
- Willing to share information and resources.
- A variety of clinical skills.
- Help you and your love one feel safe during a session.

Key 11
If Your Veteran Has Problems
With Anger

With PTSD, it is common to respond to all stressful situations as life-threatening.

You can't control that anger, but you can control how you respond to it.

1. SAFETY FIRST! If you feel your safety is threatened in any way, remove yourself from the situation and go somewhere safe. You may need to call for help.
2. Set clear boundaries about what you will and will not tolerate.
3. Wait until things calm down. Then calmly talk about the situation.
4. Remove yourself from the situation if your loved one does not calm down.
5. If it's difficult for you to stand up for yourself, seek counseling or therapy.

If Your Relationship Becomes Violent

In the event of an emergency, CALL 911!

For spouses and those in romantic relationships with a veteran, both men and women returning from war may be prone to acts of domestic violence. Take necessary precautions to protect yourself, especially if you have children.

- Trust your feelings. One outburst of rage or anger may indicate more of the same.
- Learn the warning signs of someone who might become controlling or violent.
- Get help. Talk with someone who specializes in domestic and intimate partner violence.

If your Soldier, Sailor, Airman, or Marine affected by PTSD becomes controlling or abusive, you must get help immediately! Abusive or violent relationships get worse over time.

In the event of an emergency, CALL 911!

Key 12
Approach Addiction Issues With Ease

Though not all veterans will experience substance addiction, veterans may turn to alcohol or drugs for various reasons. There is no magic formula to help someone stop drinking or drug use; however there are some things you can do:

1. Learn as much as you can about alcoholism and drug dependence. The more you know, the better you'll be able to help.
2. Speak with your veteran about your concerns, and offer your help and support, including your willingness to go with them to get help.
3. Express love and concern. Don't wait for your loved one to hit rock bottom before voicing your concerns.
4. Don't expect them to stop without help.
5. Support recovery as an ongoing process. Sobriety is NOT an event with an end in mind.

Ensure Victory By Avoiding These Pitfalls

In order to avoid defeat, steer clear of the
following:

- Preaching. Don't lecture, threaten, bribe,
  sermonize or moralize.
- Martyrdom. Avoid emotional appeals
  that may only increase feelings of guilt
  and the compulsion to drink or use other
  drugs.
- Denial… Don't cover up, lie or make
  excuses for your veteran and their
  behavior.
- Inappropriately accepting responsibility.
  Don't take on their stuff. Taking over
  responsibilities prevents another to
  accept the consequences of their
  behavior.
- Avoid arguing with them when they're
  drunk or high.
- Let go of feeling guilty or responsible for
  your loved one's behavior.
- Avoid drinking or using yourself.

Key 13
Encourage Your Veteran To Develop
Spiritual Or Religious Practice

There are many forms of spirituality, but the most effective are those that involve community, compassion, forgiveness, self-reflection and regularity. Here's how you can gently coax your veteran to trying a church or spiritual community:

1. Invite regularly.
2. Always speak from a place of good news and love, not judging.
3. Avoid using guilt. "You're going to hell" doesn't work.
4. Promote friendship, forgiveness and meaning.
5. State that you are praying for them, not a whole group of strangers.
6. Bribery! You read that correctly! Your veteran will be more receptive to going if there's a picnic.
7. Offer options, despite your individual practice and allow them to make up their own mind. Spiritual health is an important part of ultimate victory over PTSD.

Why Spirituality Can Be Effective

"Research also indicates that healthy spirituality is often associated with lower levels of symptoms and clinical problems in some trauma populations." (www.ptsd.va.gov)

Spirituality can help overcome PTSD by:

- Reducing risk behaviors by encouraging healthy lifestyles (e.g., less drinking or smoking).
- Providing an extended support system through involvement in spiritual communities.
- Using meaning-making, or the reframing of negative experiences that enhance coping skills and ways of understanding trauma.
- Learning to relax and self-regulate through prayer and meditation.
- Providing an environment of emotional support from caring people who genuinely want to help.
- Possible financial and physical support.

Key 14
What if Your Soldier, Sailor, Airman, Or Marine Goes To Jail?

Out of every ten prisoners, one has served in the military. Symptoms may be so severe that a veteran may act in an extreme manner, and may end up in jail. If that happens, here are some things you can do:

1. Remain calm.
2. Contact the nearest VA or Vet Center and ask for a benefits counselor.
3. If your veteran must serve time for a misdemeanor, file for a VA Apportionment.
4. See a therapist. If you have children, consider seeking therapy for them as well.
5. For parents of the veteran, your son or daughter will need your emotional and spiritual support while incarcerated.
6. Notify the VA immediately if your veteran is convicted of a crime and must serve time in prison. VA Disability Compensation will be reduced, but not eliminated, if your veteran is convicted of a felony and serving a sentence of over 60 days in prison.

Preparation In Case Your Veteran Goes To Jail.

Being aware of the following can help during these difficult times:

- Prepare for economic difficulty.
- If children are involved, new arrangements with family or trusted friends must be made.
- Prepare to face stereotypes and stigma because of what happened.
- Logistical, as well as emotional, adjustments to certain events must be made (e.g. parole, when they're released, etc.).
- You'll be thoroughly searched before each jail visit.

For veterans who go to jail, your benefits will be impacted. However, whatever circumstances led you to jail, this does not mean you will no longer be eligible or able to receive benefits. Contact the nearest VA or Vet Center and ask for a benefits counselor.

Key 15
Practice, Patience And Persistence

Patience and persistence are practical characteristics to develop when dealing with your Soldier, Sailor, Airman or Marine. Stress can be relieved, and much progress can be made.

The following steps will help make developing patience and persistence more clear:

1. Find out what other families in your situation have done.
2. Expect that life will now be much more difficult, but the rewards will be worth it.
3. Don't put a time limit on recovery or healing. The goal is the process.
4. Live your life. If you make your loved one the center of your life, you may end up resenting them. Take care of yourself.
5. Get support.
6. Do what you can to reduce stress.

Congratulate Yourself

The goal of recovery is the process. True victory over post-traumatic stress is a daily goal.

- Every day you and your Soldier, Sailor, Airman or Marine get through this together is a win.
- Even a full night's sleep is a major win.

Victory over PTSD can be achieved by applying the principles we've just discussed. Patience and persistence in their applications will bring every veteran suffering from PTSD back home with every war being where it belongs...in history!

You've finished. Before you go...

Tweet/share that you finished this book.

Please star rate this book.

Reviews are solid gold to writers. Please take a few minutes to give us some itty bitty feedback.

ABOUT THE AUTHOR

Earl J. Katigbak is a Marine Corps Veteran, having served multiple deployments to Iraq and Afghanistan. After receiving his master's degree in psychology, Earl now spends his time helping veterans who have been affected by Post-traumatic Stress Disorder and other issues.

For more information about Post-Traumatic Stress Disorder and how this and other disorders affect veterans, families and communities, go to: http://www.ptsd.va.gov/public/family/helpin g-family-member.asp

Find out how you can help! If you would like to support suicide prevention for veterans, go to: www.gofund.me/gaaduvnd

Receive a FREE gift for your help.

You can contact Earl by going to: https://goo.gl/y8m6KZ

If you enjoyed this book, you might also enjoy...

- **Your Amazing Itty Bitty® Heading Home Book** – Carolyn Owens

- **Your Amazing Itty Bitty® Safety Book** – Stephen C. Carpenter

- **Your Amazing Itty Bitty® Marijuana Manual** – Kat Bohnsack

  And Many More Amazing Itty Bitty® books online...

www.ingramcontent.com/pod-product-compliance
Lightning Source LLC
Chambersburg PA
CBHW060659280326
41933CB00012B/2242